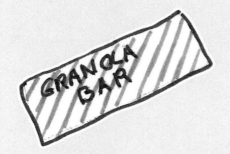

D1003903

Ava's Wish

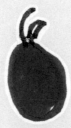

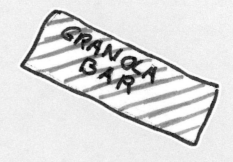

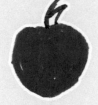

Written & Illustrated by

Millie Santilli

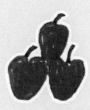

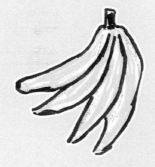

Ava's Wish. Copyright © 2020 Millie Santilli. Produced and printed by Stillwater River Publications. All rights reserved. Written and produced in the United States of America. This book may not be reproduced or sold in any form without the expressed, written permission of the author and publisher.

Visit our website at **www.StillwaterPress.com** for more information.

First Stillwater River Publications Edition

ISBN: 978-1-950339-83-9

1 2 3 4 5 6 7 8 9 10
Written & illustrated by Millie Santilli
Published by Stillwater River Publications, Pawtucket, RI, USA.

Publisher's Cataloging-In-Publication Data
(Prepared by The Donohue Group, Inc.)

Names: Santilli, Millie, author, illustrator.
Title: Ava's wish / written & illustrated by Millie Santilli.
Description: First Stillwater River Publications edition. | Pawtucket, RI, USA : Stillwater River Pub-
    lications, [2020] | Interest age level: 004-009. | Summary: "When six year-old Ava heard there
    were children who did not have enough to eat, she took upon herself to help by collecting fruit
    and healthy snacks and delivering them to her local shelter. Her wish is that all children would
    always have access to healthy foods"--Provided by publisher.
Identifiers: ISBN 9781950339839
Subjects: LCSH: Hunger--Juvenile fiction. | Homeless children--Nutrition--Juvenile fiction. | Food
    security--Juvenile fiction. | Charity--Juvenile fiction. | CYAC: Hunger--Fiction. | Homeless
    persons--Nutrition--Fiction. | Food security--Fiction. | Charity--Fiction.
Classification: LCC PZ7.1.S2638 Av 2020 | DDC [E]--dc23

The views and opinions expressed in this book are solely those of the author
and do not necessarily reflect the views and opinions of the publisher.

DEDICATIONS

This book is dedicated to John and Laura, Ava's proud parents. John and Laura have always been wonderful role models for their children. They know first hand the struggles many people face. In their early years, the two worked together at a shelter, Laura as a social worker and John as a teacher in the computer lab helping people develop new skills to get better jobs. The work was always extremely important and fulfilling to them, so it is no wonder that John and Laura would live their lives giving back any way they can, and passing that gift on to their children. Teaching by example has always been their family creed.

In this day and age when children are only looking out for what they can get for themselves, it is certaintly a true testiment of the amazing upbringing that Ava's parents continue to provide for her, her brother Jack, and her sister Lila. The world is a better place when everyone cares and wants to make a difference. Ava is on the right path and I'm sure you will be hearing a lot more about her in the future.

Ava is now 8 1/2 years old and continues going back to the shelter as often as she can. A portion of the proceeds from this book will help Ava continue her mission. Ava hopes that someday the children she has helped will pay it forward and follow in her footsteps to continue what she has started.

This book has been written by a very proud Mimi.

When six-year-old Ava heard that there were children who didn't have enough food to eat, it made her very sad.

How could that be? Children who don't have enough food? Ava came from a family where there was always enough food and snacks for her, her brother Jack, and her sister Lila.

Ava went to bed that night and tried not think about it, but it wasn't possible. It was all she could think about. Ava got into bed and looked out her window and wished upon a star,

**"Little star up in the sky,
take my wish and make it fly!"**

Ava was determined to find a way to help. Ava's wish was for all children to have as much food as she did. Ava closed her eyes and fell asleep.

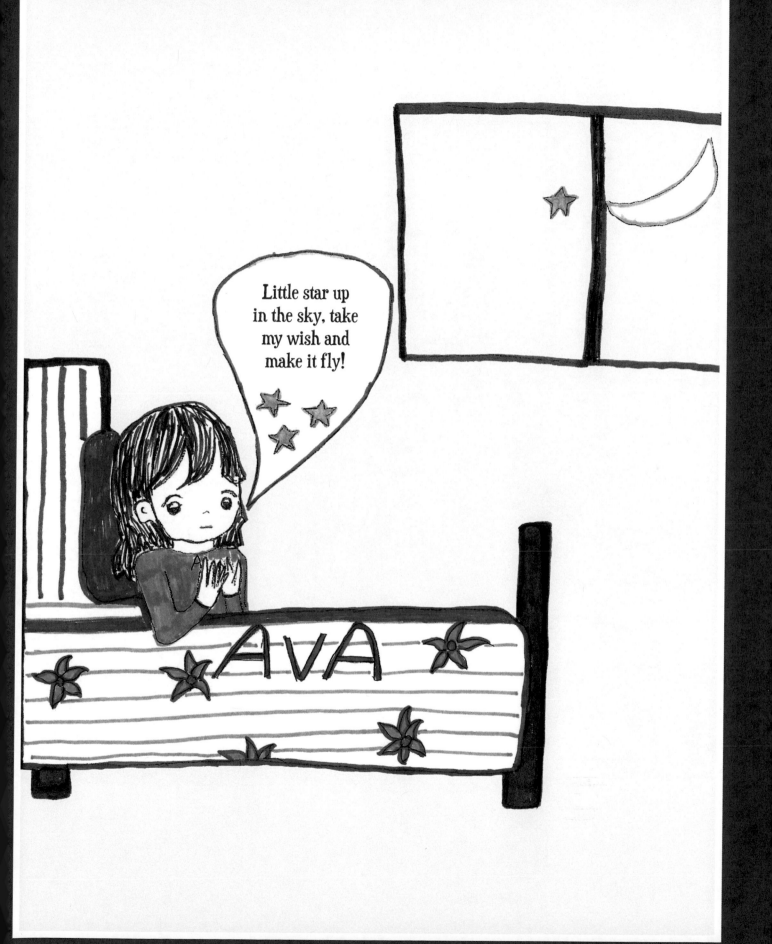

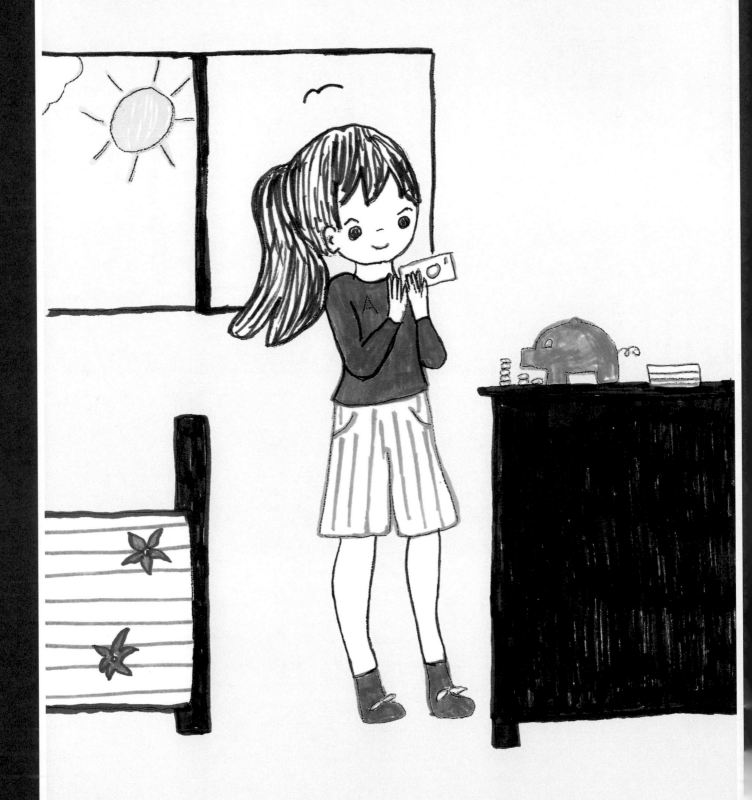

The next morning Ava talked to her mom and dad about what she wanted to do. She had an idea about taking money out of her piggy bank and then asking her mom if she would take her to buy snacks and fresh fruits to give to the children who didn't have any. Ava's mom and dad were so proud of what she wanted to do that they were very happy to take her to the market or any other place she wanted to go to buy what she needed.

Now came the hard part. Where would she go? Ava remembered that her Auntie Karen was in charge of many shelters so she asked her mom if she would call her. Ava's mom was happy to.

Auntie Karen thought it was a great idea and was so touched and proud that her young niece would be thinking of doing something like this that she went to work to find the perfect place for Ava to help.

Auntie Karen arranged for Ava to visit one of the family shelters that had many children. She knew this was just what Ava was looking for.

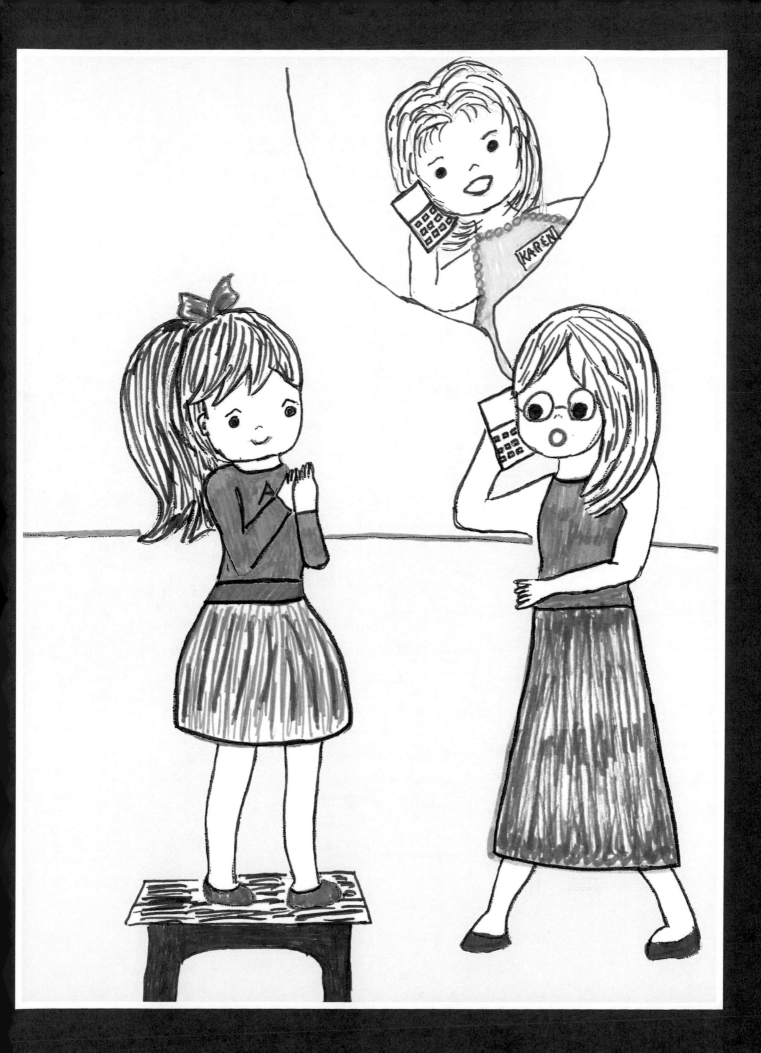

GROCERY STORE

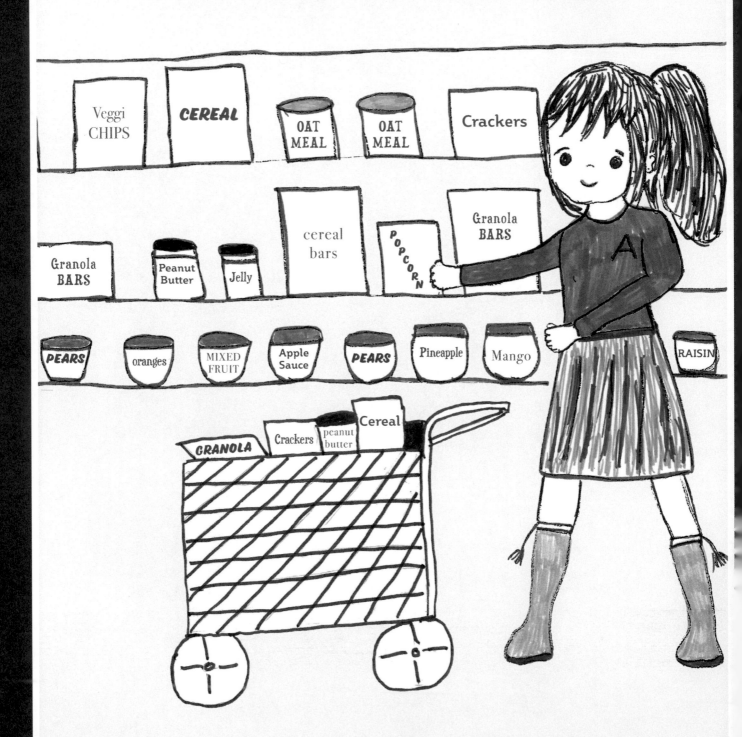

Ava's mom and dad took her to the market and watched as she walked through the store. It was as if she had been doing this forever. She carefully looked at the granola bars, applesauce, peaches—anything she thought were healthy snacks. After all, Ava's mom gave all of these snacks to her for lunch so she knew what healthy snacks were.

Then Ava moved on to the fresh fruits. Ava carefully picked out fresh strawberries, blueberries, apples, bananas, kiwi, and anything else that she thought they would like. Ava chose these items because she liked all of these fruits herself, so she was sure they would too.

The day to go to the shelter was finally here. Ava packed up all her snacks and fresh fruit, got into the car, and off they went. Ava's brother Jack and sister Lila went along to help.

As they got closer, Ava had no idea what to expect. Would they like the food she chose? Would they be friendly? Ava took a deep breath and went in to set-up her table with Jack and Lila.

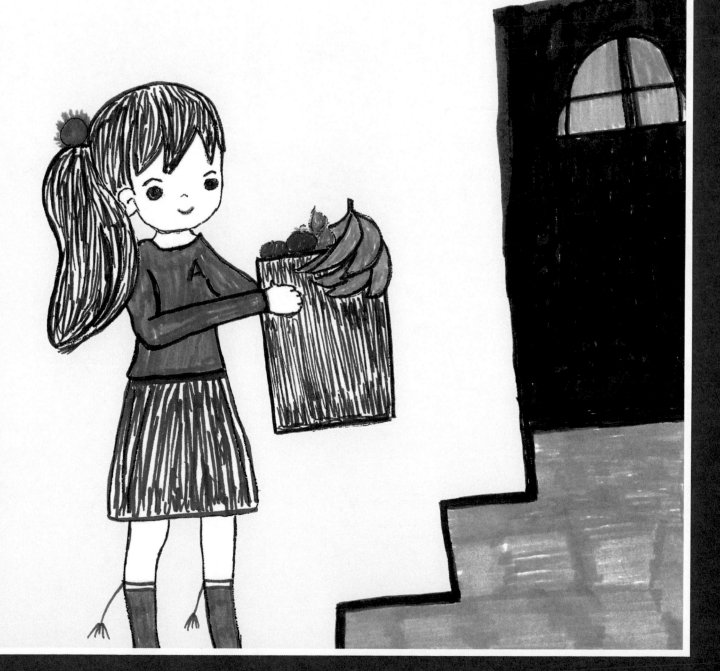

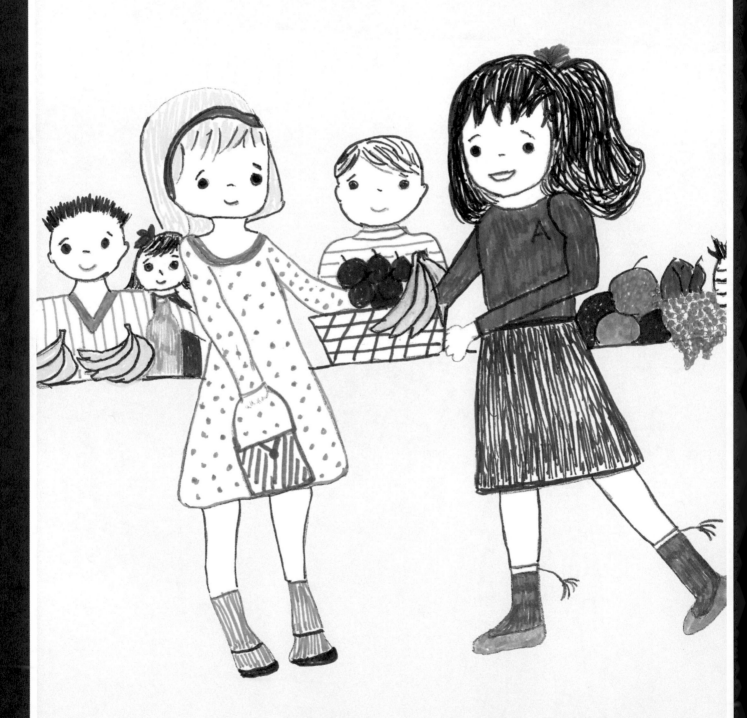

Ava was so surprised! The kids were so happy to see her and so friendly. When she put everything out on the table, they went for the fresh fruit before anything else. The children were so excited and wanted to know when she was coming back.

The day turned out better than Ava could have ever imagined. She was so happy and felt so good about helping that she decided she wanted to keep going back.

Helping people makes me happy!

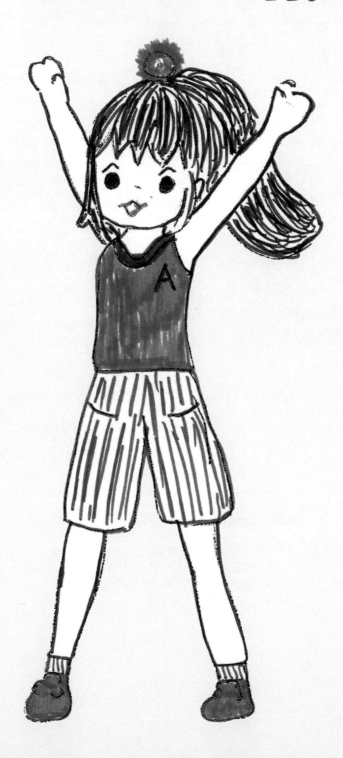

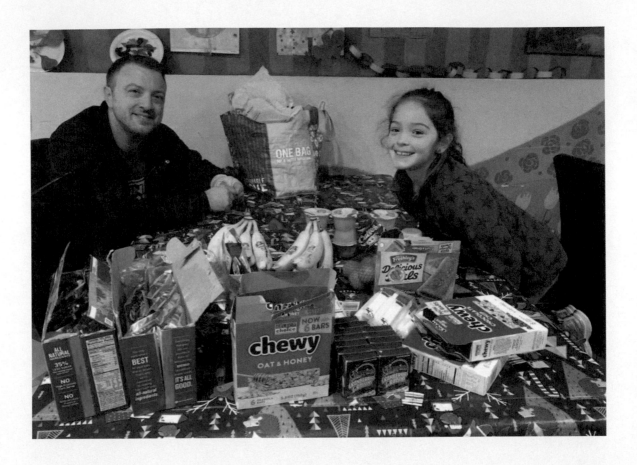

Ava's wish is to continue to go back to the shelter regularly and bring more fresh fruit and healthy snacks to the children. Ava has touched so many with her acts of kindness and her big heart that she started to receive donations from family members, the first monetary donation coming from her Uncle Louis and Auntie Colleen. Before you knew it, other family and friends wanted to donate too. Even Ava's brother Jack and sister Lila donated money from their piggy banks to help Ava.

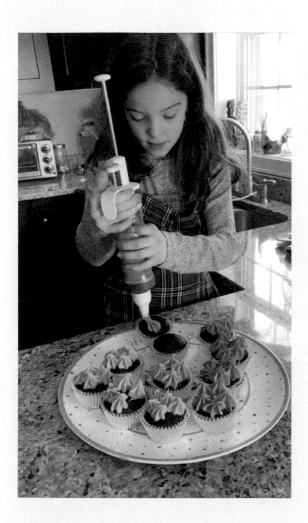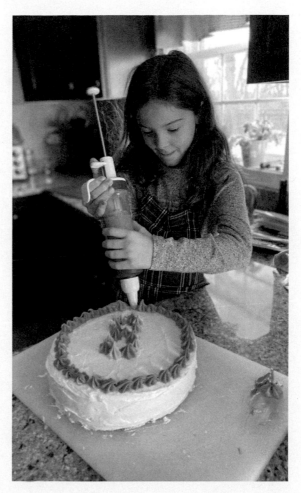

When other 6 year olds are looking to go to the playground, or ride their bikes and just have fun, Ava had something else in mind. Ava had a wish that every child would have healthy snacks and food and she was determined to find a way to make it happen. Ava's future plans are to raise money by baking homemade cupcakes and cookies and selling them for the holidays.

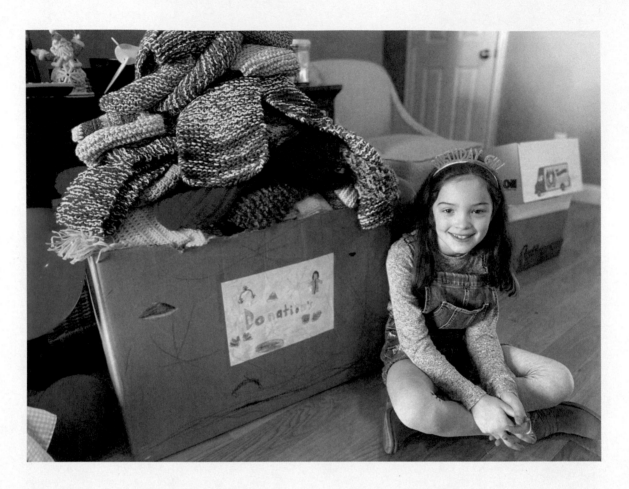

Ava's story continues on. For her 8th birthday in January, Ava expanded her mission and asked everyone to bring a clothing donation for the shelter instead of gifts for her. Ava's Vovoa's church group heard about what Ava was doing and were so touched by Ava's kindness they couldn't wait to help. The church group donated handmade knitted hats, scarves, and gloves. These generous donations were greatly appreciated not only by Ava, but also by the children at the shelter.

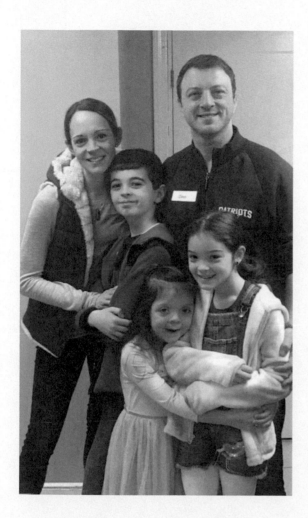 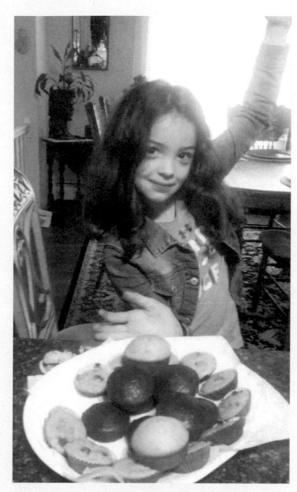

This is Ava's proud family: Mom, Dad Jack, Lila, and of course, Ava

Ava also received monetary donations from family members that will help her continue her visits to the shelter. Ava's wish is to help children who are less fortunate than she is, and she wants to challenge other kids to do the same. Ava is asking for other kids to think about organizing something in their own communities.

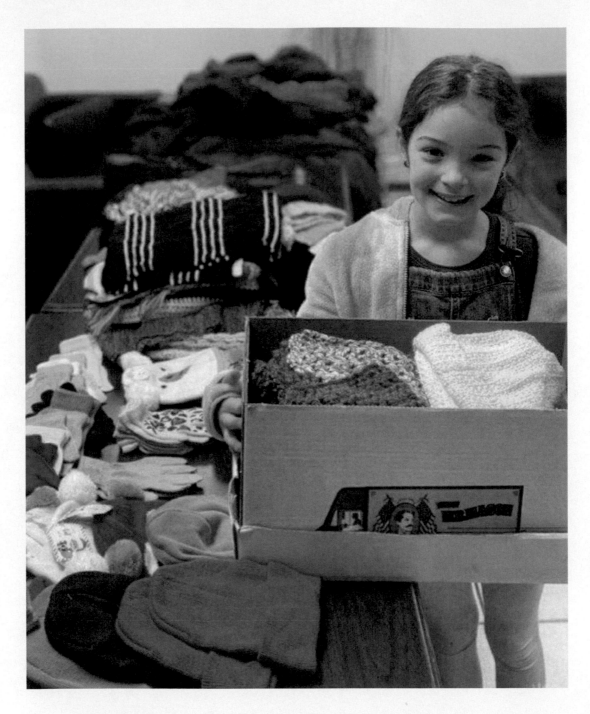

Ava's Mimi wants everyone to know that all it takes is one exceptional little girl with a wish, a mission, and a very big heart to make a difference. Watch out world, here she comes!!!

ABOUT THE AUTHOR

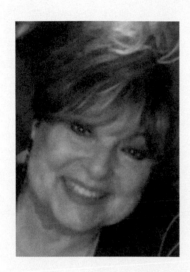

This is Millie's second children's book, the first titled *Lila Lu and the Things I Love to Do*. Millie finds inspiration from her everyday life and the people in it. Ava's wish is a true story about Millie's granddaughter, proving that one little girl's wish and determination can make anything possible. Watch for more inspirational children's books from Millie in the near future.

ILLUSTRATIONS WERE INSPIRED BY AVA SANTILLI

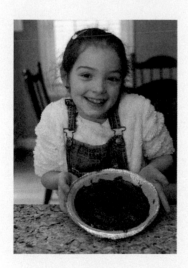

Ava's creativity was challenged when she took what she knew about the book and came up with drawings of what she thought the pages should look like, then gave them to her Mimi who drew the illistrations from her ideas, bringing the pages to life. Once again proving what an exceptional little girl Ava is, always hands on and willing to help in every way she can.

Made in the USA
Middletown, DE
24 July 2020

12353934R10015